Paleo SIMPLIFIED: Create Tasty Paleo Meals in No Time with 3 or Fewer Ingredients

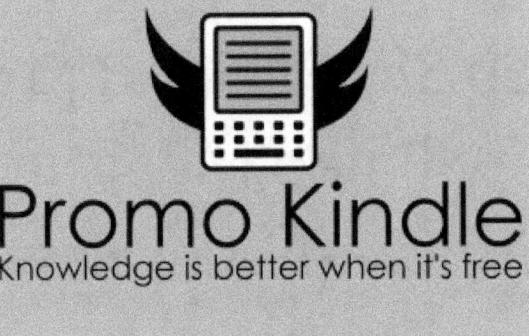

Disclaimer and Terms of Use: Effort has been made to ensure that the information in this book is accurate and complete, however, the author and the publisher do not warrant the accuracy of the information, text and graphics contained within the book due to the rapidly changing nature of science, research, known and unknown facts and internet. The Author and the publisher do not hold any responsibility for errors, omissions or contrary interpretation of the subject matter herein. This book is presented solely for motivational and informational purposes only.

Table of Contents

Cauliflower Wraps

Ingredients:
- ½ head cauliflower, cut up
- 2 eggs
- ½ tsp. curry powder
- ¼ tsp salt

Directions:

I. Start with preheating your oven to 350 degrees and lining our baking dish

II. Add your cauliflower to a food processor or blender and blend until in a chunky dry like texture

III. Add water, and crumbs in a saucepan and cook on medium for around 8-10 minutes

IV. Drain the cauliflower, and add this to a bowl with an other ingredients.

V. Form dough into two small circles, and bake on parchment paper for 15-17 minutes

Frozen Bananas

Ingredients:
- 3 bananas, ripe and sliced
- ¼ C peanut butter
- 1 bag chocolate chips

Directions:

I. Slice your bananas and place them in rows on parchment paper lined baking dish, add peanut butter on top of each banana

II. Top the peanut buttered banana's with another banana slice

III. Melt your chocolate chips in a microwave safe bowl

IV. Dip the banana with peanut butters in the chocolate and place back on parchment paper

V. Add baking sheets to freezer and let chocolate harden

VI. Serve

Ginger Berry Sorbet

Ingredients:

- 2 banana's
- 1 C frozen strawberries
- 1 tsp. grated ginger

Directions:

I.   Add everything to your blender and blend until smooth
II.   You can serve right away or blend and freeze for later

Homemade Mayonnaise

Ingredients:
- ½ C coconut butter
- ½ C warm water
- ¼ C EVOO
- 4 T minced garlic
- ¼ tsp raw salt

Directions:

I. Add everything together in our blender and blend on high, but you want to make sure that the sauce is thick.

II. Let sit and cool for about an hour

III. Refrigerate what you don't use

Seafood Peppers

Ingredients:
- Bell peppers
- Canned tuna, drained
- Homemade Mayo

Directions:

I.   Preheat your oven to 350 degrees
II.   Slice top off of your peppers.
III.   Mix your homemade mayo with the tuna
IV.   Stuff tuna mix into the peppers and bake for 25 minutes
V.   Serve

Turkey Tacos

Ingredients:
- 1 lbs. ground turkey ¼ C water
- 2 tsp taco seasoning

Directions:

I.   Cook your ground turkey on medium heat over a skillet,
II.   Once turkey is cooked, add water and seasoning
III.   Stir well, and continue to simmer

Empanadas

Ingredients:
- 1 lbs. chicken breast
- ¼ C salsa
- 1 pkt. Pillsbury Crescent rolls (yes they are Paleo friendly)

Directions:

I.   Cook our chicken breast in a skillet, shredding your meat, once cooked, stir in your Paleo salsa

II.   Preheat your oven to 350 degrees

III.   Roll out the crescent rolls, and stuff each triangle with the chicken salsa mix, roll and close each one up

IV.   Bake for 10-12 minutes

V.   Serve

Paleo Caramel Sauce

Ingredients:
- ½ C coconut milk
- ¼ C raw honey
- 2 T EVOO

Directions:

I. Add everything together in a small saucepan on high heat
II. Whisk consistently to make sure no burning or sticking on bottom of your pan
III. When reaches boil, power heat but KEEP WHISKING
IV. Once thickens, lower heat to lowest setting
V. When it reaches a nice golden brown, its done

Homemade Hazelnut

Ingredients:
- 2+2 raw almonds
- 2 C raw hazelnuts
- ½ tsp Himalayan salt
- 2 Vanilla beans

Directions:

I.   Start with preheating your oven to 350 degrees
II.   Add 2 C of almonds and 2 C hazelnuts to your baking sheet and toast for 12 minutes
III.   Move the nuts to a dish towel and wrap up to keep warm
IV.   Add everything to a blender or food processor and blend well, for 20 minutes
V.   Pour into an air tight container

Paleo Turtles

Ingredients:

- 4-5 dates, pitted and soaked
- 4 T raw pecans, crushed
- 1/3 C dark chocolate chips, vegan
- ½ tsp coconut oil

Directions:

I. Melt your chocolate in a microwave safe boil with the oil and set aside
II. Press pecan crumbs into the dates
III. Dip the dates into your chocolate and line them up along parchment paper
IV. Once all dates are dipped chocolate, set paper in freezer or plate or baking sheet to let the chocolate set.

Paleo Breakfast

Ingredients:

- ½ C coconut milk
- 3 T coconut flour
- W T shredded coconut
- ½ banana

Directions:

I.   Mix your liquids in a bowl and add shredded coconut
II.   Bring to a steady boil and whisk in the mashed banana

Fruit Cake

Ingredients:
- 1 Seedless watermelon
- 2 C coconut milk
- 1/2tsp vanilla + 1T raw honey
- 1 C sliced almonds to garnish

Whipped Cream

Directions:
I.   Start with the creamed, add the coconut to the fridge for around 6 hours, minimum

II.   Scrape out the cream and add to a bowl, add the vanilla and hone and whip, b hand or hand mixer. You want this light and fluffy.

Toasted almonds

I.   Heat skillet over medium heat and add the shredded coconut and any almonds and toast lightly

II.   Slice your watermelon by removing the top and bottom of the watermelon and the rind from the middle

III.   You want a cake shaped watermelon

IV.   Slice your watermelon into cake slice, or however you want to serve the watermelon

V.   Take one slice at a time and dip into the whipped cream coconut mixture

VI.   Then the almonds

VII.   Reassemble the cake with each piece as our dip it

Paleo Cups

Ingredients:

- ¼ C cocoa powder
- ¼ C coconut oil
- 2 T raw honey

Directions:

I.   In a saucepan whisk together the ingredients until smooth over low heat. You want this thick
II.   Line your muffin tins, and coat cupcakes
III.   Freeze in freezer until hard

Tulsa Glee

Ingredients:
- 4 C brewed Tulsi tea
- 3 T grass fed Gelatin
- 2 T raw honey

Directions:

I.   Whisk together the tea and gelatin
II.   Let this mixture set for about 5 minutes
III. Add heat, and whisk until your gelatin melts or dissolves
IV.   Let cool at room temperature and whisk in your honey
V.   Pour in a mold and let chill and set

Pumpkin Flats

Ingredients:
- 2 eggs
- ¼ C pumpkin puree
- 1/8 tsp. cinnamon

Directions:

I.   Heat your skillet and coat with a little butter or oil

II.   Whisk together your pancake batter, and add ½ to 1 C batter to skillet and make pancakes

III.   Cook on each side, flipping when necessary

Snack Caramel Apples

Ingredients:
- 1 C honey
- 1 C coconut cream
- Apples

Directions:

I. Stir your ingredients together and whisk well

II. Make sure you have a candy thermometer handy

III. Heat until reaches 245 degrees, let it start to bubble. This can take up to half an hour

IV. When caramel is ready, add skewers to your apples and dip apples into caramel

V. Add parchment paper to sheet or plate and add your caramel dipped apples to the paper and let set

Crunchy Banana Snack (Single serve)

Ingredients:
- 1 banana
- 3 T nuts and seeds

Directions:

I.   Start with peeling the banana and laying out on a baking dish

II.   Sprinkle nuts and seeds or roll banana in the seeds

III.   This is a single serve recipes, just repeat for each banana

Plantain Waffles

Ingredients:

- 1 yellow plantain
- 1 egg
- ¼ tsp baking soda

Directions:

I.   Peel and puree the plantain
II.   Add in rest of ingredients and whisk well
III. Use waffle iron to make waffles

Pesto Sauce

Ingredients:
- 1 avocado
- ½ C basil + ½ tsp minced garlic
- 1 ½ T lemon juice

Directions:

I.   Add everything in for food processor, blend until basil is crushed
II.   Add in peel or flesh of avocado, and blend.
III.   Store in cold fridge

Banana Custard

Ingredients:
- 3 eggs
- 2 bananas
- 1 C coconut milk

Directions:

I. Star with preheating your oven to 350 degrees
II. Add your ingredients to a small mixing bowl whisk together briefly then pour into food processor or blender and blend
III. Divide the blended custard into mason jars or serving bowls
IV. Bake for 45 minutes
V. Cool and refrigerate

Espresso Cakes

Ingredients:
- 2 bananas
- 2 eggs
- 1 T ground espresso beans

Directions:
I.   Heat your skillet with a little oil in the pan
II.   Mash bananas and whisk in the eggs and espresso beans
III.   Whisk batter, and use about ¼ C per pancake
IV.   Heat and flip

Coconut yogurt

Ingredients:
- 4 C coconut milk
- 1 T sweetener
- Yogurt starter

Directions:

I.   Heat the milk and sweetener, and bring to a slow boil

II.   You want this to reach 115 degrees, you need to use a candy thermometer if needed

III.   Add in the starter powder and stir well

IV.   Cover and let sit in dark oven for at least 8 hours

Homemade coconut milk

Ingredients:
- 2 C shredded organic coconut
- 4 C boiling water

Directions:

I.   Pour boiling water over shredded coconut and let sit for around 30 minutes
II.   Pour this mixture into the blender and blend until smooth
III.   Strain the coconut and save milk and refrigerate.

www.ingramcontent.com/pod-product-compliance
Lightning Source LLC
Chambersburg PA
CBHW071349310526
45790CB00018B/1399